DEDICATION

I dedicate this book to my family especially to my husband. He never fails to understand my everyday shortcomings. I also dedicated this book to my loving son who is my riding buddy.

TABLE OF CONTENTS

Arthritis Cure: Natural Ways to Beat Arthritis

Have a Pain Free Life Even with Arthritis

By: Judith Peters

9781634289931

PUBLISHERS NOTES

Disclaimer – Speedy Publishing LLC

This publication is intended to provide helpful and informative material. It is not intended to diagnose, treat, cure, or prevent any health problem or condition, nor is intended to replace the advice of a physician. No action should be taken solely on the contents of this book. Always consult your physician or qualified health-care professional on any matters regarding your health and before adopting any suggestions in this book or drawing inferences from it.

The author and publisher specifically disclaim all responsibility for any liability, loss or risk, personal or otherwise, which is incurred as a consequence, directly or indirectly, from the use or application of any contents of this book.

Any and all product names referenced within this book are the trademarks of their respective owners. None of these owners have sponsored, authorized, endorsed, or approved this book.

Always read all information provided by the manufacturers' product labels before using their products. The author and publisher are not responsible for claims made by manufacturers.

This book was originally printed before 2014. This is an adapted reprint by Speedy Publishing LLC with newly updated content designed to help readers with much more accurate and timely information and data.

Speedy Publishing LLC

40 E Main Street, Newark, Delaware, 19711

Contact Us: 1-888-248-4521

Website: http://www.speedypublishing.co

REPRINTED Paperback Edition: ISBN: 9781634289931

Manufactured in the United States of America

Chapter 1 - Get to Know Arthritis More

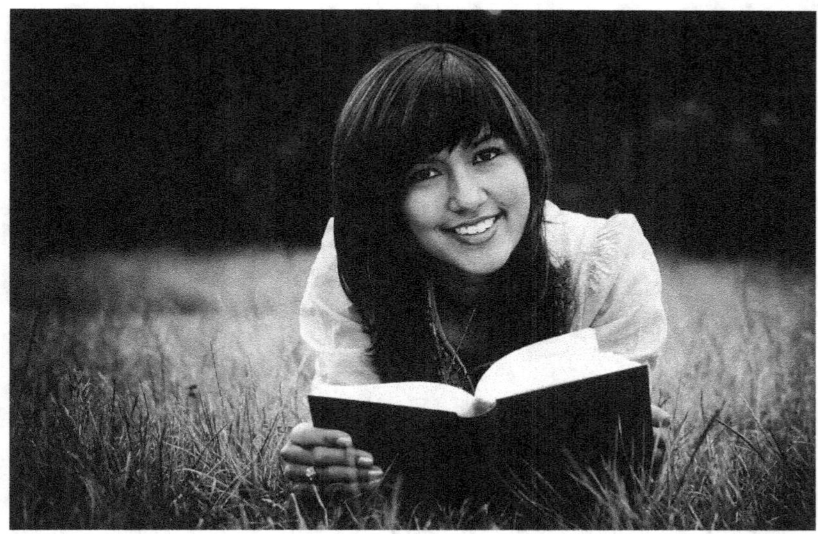

When you hear the word arthritis, images of painful hands and joints comes into play. Few people fully understand arthritis and this guide is dedicated to anyone suffering with this chronic condition and wants relief now.

Rheumatoid arthritis is known to be an autoimmune disease. Inflammation of the synovium causes chemicals to thicken the thin layer of tissue which lines and lubricates the joint.

The thickened synovium may eventually damage the cartilage and ultimately the bone. Arthritics suffering with RA may experience symptoms, such as pain, stiffness, swelling and impaired function of the affected joint. In advanced cases the condition may lead to configuration and twisting of the affected area.

Rheumatoid arthritis can be apparent in any age and is not confined to one sex, having said that RA does tend to be more prevalent in females; women are thought to be three times more likely to suffer with rheumatoid arthritis than men.

RA is not often restricted to just one joint, many arthritics will often find themselves symmetrically affected, such as in both hands, or perhaps in both knees. People have suffered with arthritis since the dawn of time itself; however the condition has become far more common in our recent past.

Arthritis along with numerous other conditions is now so common, they could almost be labeled as diseases of our time, and our modern world has accelerated our poor health.

Tens of millions are reported to be afflicted with one type of arthritis or another, while millions more suffer in silence. The number of known cases of arthritis has almost doubled in the last 20 years, and only seems to gather to gather momentum by the day.

It's estimated that one in three of us will experience symptoms of arthritis to some degree, at some point in our lives. This terrible disease shows no sign of slowing, & some experts have reportedly gone as far as saying that future generations may all be affected by arthritis to some degree.

Statistics from the Centers for Disease Control estimates that if numbers continue to rise, very soon, one out of four adults will suffer from the disease at some point during their life. Currently the estimates are as high as 70 MILLION Americans suffering from arthritis.

Arthritis has in the past been mistakenly labeled as a consequence of ageing, and while it is true that this disease is far more common amongst the older population, we now know arthritis is not linked only to age. Men, women, children even animals are susceptible to this debilitating disease, there are no exceptions and the reasons could be right under our noses.

It's a growing belief among many that arthritis, especially Rheumatoid Arthritis is a symptom of the body's intolerance to certain toxins & environmental pollutants. Perhaps this sounds very complicated and unavoidable?

The truth is that these toxins may not be what you expect them to be. Throughout this book I will attempt to uncover the real reason you suffer with Rheumatoid Arthritis & more importantly how you can reverse the symptoms in weeks without medication.

While there are many different varieties of the disease, the term "arthritis" has been used to describe in a much broader sense anyone suffering joint and chronic mobility pain, joint swelling, as well as overall stiffness.

There also appears to be no end in sight to the explosive growth of people that are contracting arthritis at an earlier age. Because arthritis is primarily an autoimmune disease, many people are susceptible to contracting arthritis.

New studies link decreased nutrition and all forms of toxins that are invading our food chain as contributing to the body's immune system breaking down and mistakenly attacking joints, cartilage and other areas of the body.

Other diseases and events in your life can contribute to contracting arthritis; such as bacterial infections, gout even medical treatments that can affect your cartilage can become issues that later develop into full blown arthritis.

While we could go into great detail about the specifics of each different kinds of arthritis our main concern is the pattern of severity and locations of where arthritis in a general term seems to occur in the human body and how to reverse this naturally.

CHAPTER 2- DIFFERENT TYPES OF ARTHRITIS THAT YOU SHOULD KNOW

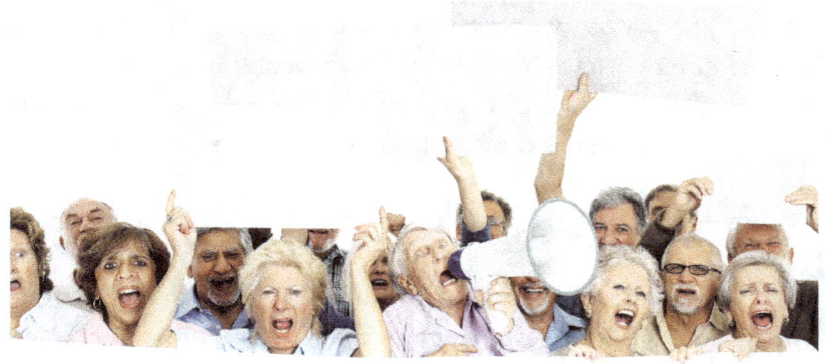

There are currently more than 100 types of arthritis, which affect more than 46 million adults in the US alone. Symptoms can vary from person to person, depending on what type of arthritis you have.

Arthritis can affect your entire body and can be caused by a number of different factors. Many arthritis symptoms are common in all types of arthritis however; there are differences you should be aware of.

To name a few, here are the different common types of arthritis and their symptoms.

Osteoarthritis

This is the most common form in older people. It is caused mostly by long-term everyday use. Depending on which part of the body is affected, symptoms may vary and include pain, swelling and inflammation. Most people with osteoarthritis in their fingers don't even realize they have it unless an x-ray reveals the deterioration in their cartilage. Osteoarthritis never goes away, however the pain can be managed and is usually only noticed during flare-ups.

Rheumatoid

This type of arthritis is caused by an overactive immune system. The symptoms usually start out as minor pain and stiffness and may come and go at first. Over time, flare-ups become more frequent and painful. Treatment for this type of arthritis is most effective when started within the first few months showing symptoms.

Bursitis

This form of arthritis usually affects the hip, shoulder, and elbow. However, it can also affect the knee, heel, or base of big toe. Usually this affects athletes, golfers, baseball players, or people who are out of shape and have poor posture. Its symptoms are pain soreness and stiffness in the joint and become worse when joint is used. The joint may also be swollen and warm to the touch.

Gout

Many people don't realize that gout is a form of arthritis and occurs where the body has too much uric acid. The symptoms of gout are intense pain in the joint (usually the big toe). It may also become red, swollen, and warm to the touch. It can also occur in the wrists, ankles, and knees. Symptoms are only noticeable during flare-ups and may not come back for several years, but if crystals formed by the uric acid are left untreated, it can actually destroy bone.

Ankylosing spondylitis

This is arthritis of the joints in the spine also known as MarieStrumpell disease and rheumatoid spondylitis. This disorder affects multiple organs such as eyes, heart, lungs, skin, and gastrointestinal tract. Symptoms include lower back and hip pain, stiffness, difficulty expanding the chest, pain in the neck, shoulders, knees, and ankles. Sufferers can also experience fatigue, weight loss and run low-grade fever. Symptoms with this type of arthritis are often uncommon after the age of 30, although many patients aren't diagnosed before then.

Juvenile

Many people associate arthritis with the elderly. However, according to Arthritis Foundation, one out of every 250 children under the age of 18 suffers from this disease. Its symptoms are similar to adult sufferers and include pain, swelling, and joint stiffness. The symptoms can come and go and especially in cases of young children, they don't complain about their pain. Parents may not notice there is a problem until they see their child limping, avoiding physical activity, or displaying unusual clumsiness.

When you are experiencing any signs of arthritis symptoms, you should contact your doctor and see a proper diagnosis because treatment is always more effective when this disease is caught in the early stages.

Chapter 3- Most Common Causes of Arthritis

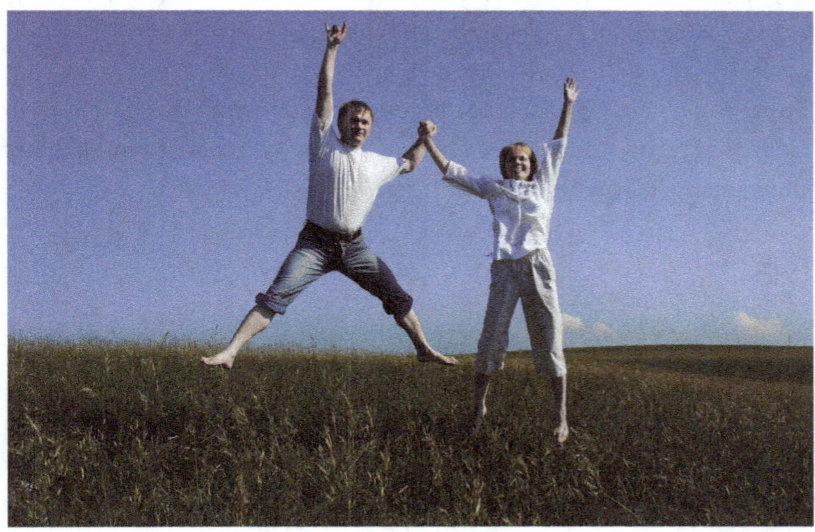

Many factors are known to contribute towards different types of arthritis, unfortunately even with modern day medical practices, identifying any specific route cause is almost impossible which makes effective treatment difficult.

Listed within this chapter are some widely accepted risk factors, and causes which are known to contribute towards all types of arthritis. Also listed are some lesser known possibility's which research indicates may also having a bearing.

This is just a small list of some of the risk factors thought to be responsible for and attributed to arthritis, many prescribed and over the counter drugs may also play a very damaging part which we will cover later.

OBESITY

Excess weight puts unnecessary pressure on the supporting joints, especially hips and knees. It is hard to say whether obesity actually causes arthritis, or if having arthritis leads to obesity.

Either way obesity has a detrimental effect on all of us. It is very clear that a reduction in weight will greatly help people in all walks of life, especially arthritics suffering with osteoarthritis.

AGE

As the body becomes older it may become more susceptible to arthritis. The reason for arthritis being more prevalent in the elderly is due mainly to the bone becoming brittle. With age, an increasingly brittle cartilage has less capacity to repair itself, which may ultimately lead to arthritis.

A lesser known reason for rheumatoid arthritis becoming worse or developing with age may be a buildup of toxins throughout the gastrointestinal tract.

PREVIOUS INJURY / TRAUMA

It is very common for osteoarthritis to develop after a serious accident, trauma even surgery. Osteoarthritis will frequently develop in the joint where the damage occurred.

SEX

Arthritis, as we know, is not a disease restricted to sex, however woman are far more likely to develop arthritis, especially rheumatoid arthritis. Research has suggested a figure of around 60% of all arthritics to be female.

Gout tends to be more prevalent in the male population, articles linked to grout suggest alcohol may be a contributing factor & may help explain why more men than women suffer with this condition.

GENETICS / FAMILY

Studies into the causes of arthritis suggest the association of specific genes which could be linked to certain types of arthritic conditions.

It's thought that rheumatoid arthritis or genes containing the disease may be passed down through family generations.

Having the gene passed to you through family puts you at a higher risk of developing arthritis, known as genetic predisposition; this however does not mean you will develop the condition.

SMOKING

Smoking cigarettes and passive smoking has damaging effects on many parts of the human body; it's clear to everyone what smoking does to their heart and lungs, not to mention their skin.

You may be surprised to learn that studies now indicate a very strong link between smoking and rheumatoid arthritis. The connection is yet to be fully understood, but research has shown that smoking releases excess free radicals and toxins into the bloodstream.

Excess free radicals along with numerous other toxins are known to attack and affect the immune system, which may cause abnormality in white blood cells. Smoking over a long period may also have a significant effect on bone and the bones ability to repair itself.

ALLERGIES / FOOD INTOLERENCIES

There are very few foods which cause obvious allergic reactions, the best known are probably peanuts.

Not knowing what foods you may be allergic to is a real problem, a bigger problem than you might imagine.

Many people go through life with food intolerances and never show any classical signs of an allergy, for this reason they may never suspect their favorite food may be the cause of their arthritis.

Symptoms of food intolerances, when apparent are more often than not delayed reactions, so even if you do display symptoms it can still be difficult to link a reaction with a particular food.

Nutritionists specializing in food intolerances and arthritis suggest that the main culprit will be our favorite food or beverage, the foods we crave the food or drink you can't live without. These foods may have an addictive quality.

CANDIDIASIS

Candida is normally harmless yeast contained within the gastrointestinal tract, under normal circumstances Candida is a sugar fermenting yeast which along with other micro organisms helps break down and digest food. The human body's biochemistry is very fragile and may be easily thrown off balance.

Candida can transform itself from part of the body's natural yeast, into a pathogenic fungus, a condition known as candidiasis. The transformation of Candida into candidiasis can be caused by the prolonged use of antibiotics, stress, diabetes, acidic pH level, & depleted immune system.

Candidias is growth can affect the normal functioning of the gut, without treatment the fungus can penetrate the wall of the gut causing leaky gut syndrome. Once through the wall candidiasis can pass through the bloodstream releasing toxins which can attack any of the body's organs.

Candidiasis is also known to decrease the body's nutrient uptake, leading to vitamin and mineral deficiency.

HEAVY METAL POISONING / METAL TOXICITIES

Heavy metal poisoning has become a major health problem in recent history and will inevitably become much worse, as more countries become industrialized nations. Metals and industrial bi products seep into the water and enter the food chain.

Heavy metals have a density of over five times that of water, the human body is unable to successfully break down the foreign bodies and is forced to retain them.

The accumulation of heavy metals trapped in the body causes toxicity to poison the bloodstream, leading to damaged kidneys, lungs, nervous system and other organs.

YOUR ARTHRITIS MEDICATION IS MAKING YOU WORSE...

The most common medication used to treat arthritis, are Anti-inflammatory, Steroids & Non-Steroid Anti-inflammatory, along with the more aggressive treatments programs. The problem with prescribed and over the counter drugs used to treat arthritis is at best they only mask the disease, with a temporary relief of the symptoms.

Arthritis is prevalent for a reason and has a cause, while the root cause in any specific case of arthritis is basically impossible to pinpoint, I think it unwise to tackle only the symptoms of the disease.

Treating the symptoms with drugs such as Aspirin, Ibuprofen and more aggressive drugs will over time release toxins and chemicals into the bloodstream, which may in fact be worsening the condition along with causing numerous other medical problems.

NSAIDs

NSAIDs provides only symptomatic relief and have been shown to suppress bone repair and have toxic effects on cartilage metabolism, so as with most of the drugs prescribed to treat your arthritis pain, the drug will actually damage the effected cartilage further and ultimately destroy the joint. Other side effects are known to be, Kidney failure, Liver dysfunction, Bleeding, and Gastric ulceration.

Cortisone has many other undesirable side effects, such as an impaired ability for the body to kill foreign bodies in the blood, leaving the body defenseless and open too infection

More aggressive drugs

Which may include azathioprine, methotrexate, cyclophosphamide, penicillamine and droxychloroquine that may be administered together with NSAIDs and corticosteroids? A recent study evaluated over 100 arthritic patients who were on such aggressive drug therapy over a 20year period. The results proved alarming as over one third had died and Just 18% were able to carry on their normal lives.

Chapter 4- How to Live with Arthritis

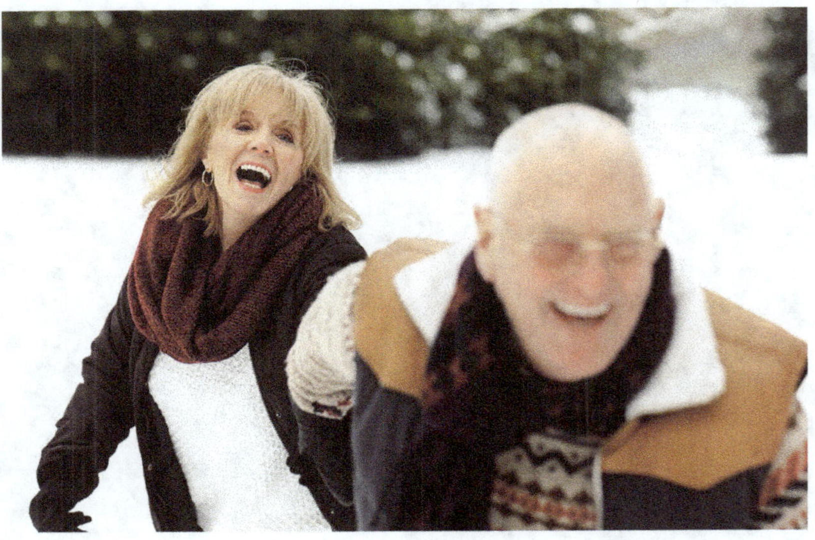

Anyone who suffers from arthritis knows it can fill your life with both physical and emotional pain. Not only does it restrict your movement, it can limit your freedom, because as symptoms progress it becomes increasingly difficult to perform simple tasks that used to be easy. It isn't just the swelling and stiffness in your joints that keep you from moving freely, it's the often debilitating pain that controls your life and makes you feel hopeless.

While there is no single method that works for everyone, there are things that you can do to help alleviate and sometimes eliminate your arthritis symptoms.

Consulting your physician is not just a good idea; a qualified doctor is capable of assisting you with the correct information necessary to make wise decisions when affecting exercise, lifestyle changes and finally can prescribe the correct medications to enhance or improve your condition.

Keep in mind that what works well for one person might not work at all for another. Many treatments for arthritis will only slow down or lessen its effects. As we have discussed before finding the right treatment plan can take time and testing before you find the exact regimen that works best for you and adjustments may be needed over time.

The most important thing that you can do is educate yourself. Find out what type of arthritis you have and learn all you can about it. Do research online, visit the Arthritis Foundation and don't be afraid to ask questions. Once diagnosed you should consider speaking with a doctor that specializes in arthritis treatments. Arthritis is a very serious disease, so don't ignore it and get proper treatment.

Here are some simple things you can try that should help alleviate the pain associated with mild flare-ups.

Pay attention to your posture.

It's never too late to practice good posture. Good posture helps with proper alignment and can often alleviate and even prevent painful flare-ups. This is because it takes the stress off your joints, muscles and promotes better circulation.

Lose weight

Carrying around even a few extra pounds can add stress to your joints and increase the pain you feel substantially.

Exercise regularly

Exercising is extremely important for arthritis sufferers because it increases blood flow, which helps get oxygen to your joints which and removes toxic deposits from afflicted areas. It can also improve your flexibility and build strong muscles to support your joints and reduce your pain.

Moderate exercising strengthens your joints and increases flexibility and stability. Those with rheumatoid arthritis need to refrain from exercising during flare ups. You should only exercise to the point where you feel mild discomfort. You should not feel pain.

Apply heat

Heat therapy can increase circulation and decrease inflammation. An added benefit from heat therapy is that it will reduce swelling and relaxes tight muscles, which relieves the stress and pain in your joints.

There are several different topical options available when it comes to using heat therapy including heating pads, gels and creams like Biofreeze or BenGay, which can be found at your local department store. There are also hot wraps, saunas and simply soaking in a hot bath.

Cold compresses

Cold can also bring relief from some type of arthritis pain. It decreases blood flow, which helps relieve the throbbing that can sometimes occur during flare-ups. It reduces swelling and can slow down the pain signals sent to your brain.

You can also try using heat and cold therapy together. By alternating between the two, you may experience longer lasting relief. Try applying heat to the affected area for five to ten minutes and then switch to cold.

Eat a healthy diet.

Not only will that help you maintain a healthy weight, but there are certain vitamins found in food that specifically help alleviate arthritis symptoms.

For instance, vitamin C repairs tissue, vitamin D absorbs calcium, builds bone mass, and prevents bone loss, and calcium strengthens your bones.

Don't leave the cold compresses on quite as long that heat compress and repeat this process multiple times for the best effect.

Get plenty of rest

The proper amount of sleep can play a very important role in your arthritis treatment. Having arthritis can be stressful to your body and your mind in many ways.

 Making sure that you are getting the adequate amount of rest will give your body a chance to heal itself. By resting and using some of the other methods we have discussed today, you may be able to alleviate many of your arthritis symptoms or at least make them more manageable, so that you can regain your freedom and enjoy your life.

Patients with arthritis should get at least 8 to 10 hours of sleep, so that the body has time to repair itself. Lack of sleep has a big affect on your overall health and physical well-being.

When your arthritis does flare up there are different treatments you can try to help alleviate the pain and inflammation.

Ice packs can help with swelling and inflammation, but people with circulatory problems should avoid this. You can also use a heating pad or take a hot bath or shower.

During particularly painful flare-ups may be necessary to use over-the-counter or prescribed medication. Certain types of medications can have serious side effects, so you need to weigh the pros and cons with your doctor before taking them.

Patients with severe arthritis may sometimes need to use splints, braces, canes, or walkers for stability during extreme flare-ups.

There are changes you can make in your home to living with arthritis easier. A "grabber" can help you get a can out of the cupboard or pick up laundry off the floor. Replace faucet handles that twist and round door knobs with levered handles.

Don't overdo it, while exercise is necessary to alleviate your symptoms, tiring yourself out can provoke flare ups for people with rheumatoid arthritis. So remember to take breaks and don't feel like you have to do everything in one day.

Being sedentary can also have a big impact on your arthritis symptoms. Sitting at a desk for 8 hours a day can result in stiff sore joints. If you have to sit for a long period of time be sure to take a breaks to move around and do stretches.

When it comes to living with arthritis there are things can do to alleviate and even prevent an arthritis flare up. The most important thing to remember is you're not alone and not to give up, you can find a solution that works for you.

It is also important to work closely with your doctor until you find the best treatment regimen for your symptoms. Don't be afraid to ask for help and check with your local Arthritis Foundation to see what resources are available to you.

CHAPTER 5- MAKE A COMPLETE PLANE TO DEAL WITH YOUR ARTHRITIS

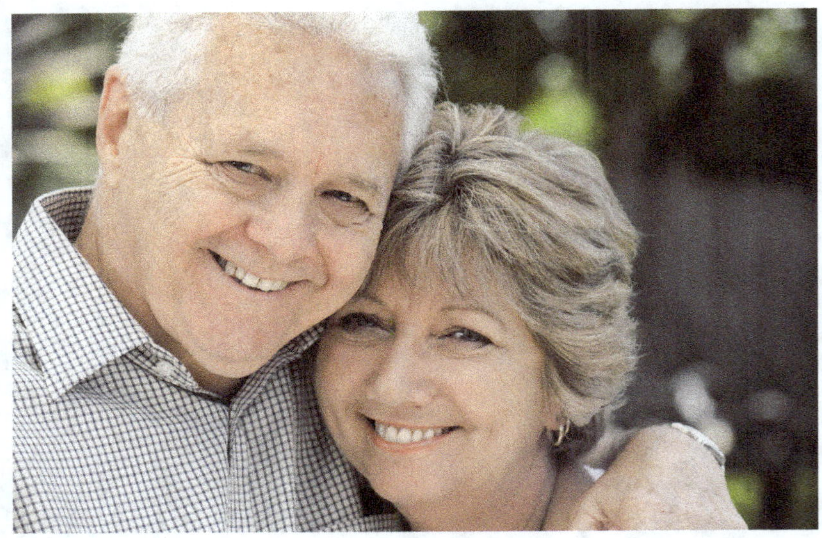

The people that have the most success in dealing with their arthritis approach their treatment from a systematic plan that incorporates different methodologies. Over time you will be able to fine tune some of the steps and each one can have a direct benefit on how you feel, reduce pain and swelling, pain management and finally greatly relieve your symptoms:

1. Consult The Right Physician while there is a general mistrust of doctors growing in America, an informed physician is your best ally when creating and maintaining a treatment plan. It is critical that you speak with a professional to evaluate your treatment to ensure you are not going to do something to further aggravate your condition.

Consulting your physician is not just a good idea; a qualified doctor is capable of assisting you with the correct information necessary to make wise decisions when affecting exercise, lifestyle changes and finally can prescribe the correct medications to enhance or improve your condition.

This does not mean however that all physicians can be of help when dealing with your arthritis. You should look for someone that specializes in geriatrics and has the ability to understand and comprehend that you wish to treat your arthritis with more than just drugs.

Several studies show that improvement in arthritis can happen simply with proper lifestyle changes and improving the quality and content of the food that you eat as well as using good mineral and vitamin supplementation.

You should approach arthritis from a chronic disease management model. Because arthritis can flare-up and cause pain and reduced mobility and then vanish, is important that our lifestyle changes take this into consideration and give our bodies the necessary nutrients in order to directly combat these occurrences.

The physician that you choose should have deep knowledge of nutrition; unfortunately most doctors that graduate from medical school today have virtually no formal education in nutrition.

You may wish to consult a professional that has a background in healing people through nutrition first as this kind of expert is precisely what is needed for helping you to deal with reducing flare ups and improving overall bodily health.

2. Incorporate Appropriate Physical Exercise regardless of your age you can benefit from additional physical exercise. You should consult a physical therapist as far as range of motion exercises to improve your arthritis. Weights bearing activities, tai chi and yoga have all been shown to drastically improve. Health conditions for

people suffering from arthritis as well as adding improved flexibility.

Even though arthritis can be very painful and discourage you from wanting to do physical exercise, there is a direct link to the amount of physical exercise that you perform and the reduction and management of your arthritis.

If you are not already consulting a physical therapist we highly recommend that you do so as well as your physician before starting any form of exercise.

A physical therapist is important because they study range of motion, and fully understand your capabilities based on tests they can administer. They can guide you on exactly the kind of exercise that you should be doing and a therapist can help manage physical limitations so as to ensure that you do not injure yourself when starting an exercise regimen.

Exercises like yoga have been shown to dramatically improve people's overall flexibility, breathing, strength and mental clarity. The nice thing about yoga is that regardless of your current health conditions you can benefit from this exercise and continue to do so at your own pace.

A beginner's yoga video can get you started and you can take your time and improve all physical aspects of your body. There is also a connection with yoga that involves deeper meditation that helps with pain management, overall feelings of wellbeing and reduced stress.

Regardless of the type of exercise that you and your physical therapist discuss, getting started on a new and healthier you will keep your range of motion, flexibility and physical strength improving.

3. Major Healthy Changes In Diet since the majority of people suffering from arthritis is due to a degree of autoimmune disease, it is important to drastically improve the quality of the food that you are eating and to strongly consider supplementation and natural herbs and spices to enhance your overall health.

Due to the over industrialization, chemical use, and micro toxic additives of found in majority of processed foods available today, most of what people eat is almost completely depleted of minerals and natural occurring vitamins.

There have been studies that directly link reduced quality of foods, pesticides, food additives, dyes etc. to the explosion of illness and disease that is taking America and the entire world by storm.

It now takes a concerted effort to eat healthy. What used to be natural and organic has now been replaced with pseudo organic foods, GMO's, irradiated foods and a whole host of new substances that are being found that harm human health.

4. Using Specific Lifestyle Changes And Folk Treatments there are a variety of suggestions in this guide that can immediately improve the way you feel and how to manage your arthritis.

The single biggest impact to dealing effectively with arthritis is lifestyle changes tied to all of the elements we have been discussing. Since some elements of involving natural treatments will also involve lifestyle changes, we have saved this portion of the four step plan for last because it opens up into a large assortment of simple things that can be done daily, weekly and monthly to both support pain management and begin to eliminate arthritis flare-ups.

Do you think you can't put an end to your arthritis pain?

Many arthritis sufferers feel that way, like there is nothing they can do to stop the aches and pains they have to endure on a daily basis. However finding relief doesn't have to be hard, complicated or expensive. Often the small things make a big difference.

Let's go over a few simple tips that may help.

Protect your joints

This means avoiding unnecessary stress like heavy lifting or prolonged physical activity when you're in pain. You should also avoid keeping them in the same position for a prolonged period, because it will cause stiffness and inflammation. Just by maintaining a good balance of physical activity and rest throughout the day you can alleviate many of your aches, pains and stiffness.

Be sure to stretch

Stretching should be part of every arthritis sufferer's daily routine. A good stretch helps warm up muscles and prevent injuries. Limber tendons are less likely to tear. Spend just 10 minutes a day stretching your major muscle groups and you will be amazed at how much better you feel.

Keep cool

If you begin to feel overheated or your joints and muscles are burning, be sure to stop and take a break. Rest in a cool, comfortable environment. To cool down faster try spraying yourself with a mist of cool water or wrap an ice pack or cold compress in a towel and apply it to reduce arthritis pain and swelling.

Keep moving

As we have discussed before regular exercise can help reduce joint pain and stiffness and increases flexibility and muscle strength. It can also help with weight control, stress management, and make you feel better overall. The Arthritis Foundation also offers water exercise and other classes.

Get a massage.

Massage therapy can relieve your pain, soothe stiff sore muscles, and reduce inflammation and swelling. Make sure you use oil or cream on your fingers to make it gentler. Work the area for five to ten minutes a day if possible.

Keep your weight in balance.

Being overweight, even just moderately, affects your weight bearing joints and can increase the pain of arthritis. Studies have indicated that losing extra weight lowers the risk for developing osteoarthritis of the knee. Losing weight can help slow the progression of arthritis too.

Get a diagnosis.

Remember, if you are experiencing persistent symptoms like pain, stiffness, swelling for more than a week, you should see your doctor and get a proper diagnosis. Don't forget, there are more than 100 types of arthritis. It is important to get the specific diagnosis for the type of arthritis you have, so you can use the right course of treatment.

Medication

If your doctor prescribes medication make sure you follow the dosage instructions. Never stop taking your medication just because you feel better or think it is not working. Always check with your doctor first. You need to understand that it may take several days to several months for a medication to become effective.

Educate yourself

New treatments for arthritis are constantly being studied, so make sure you take the time to look for new options. Recently FDA has approved some new drugs for osteoarthritis, rheumatoid arthritis and other arthritis diseases. If feel that the current medication doesn't work well, check with your doctor about possible new options.

Keep educating yourself. It is important to learn something new about arthritis. Find some good websites online and subscribe to their newsletter if they have it. Join one of two active online arthritis communities like forums or bulletin board. Never hesitate to see your doctors and ask questions.

CHAPTER 6- TREATING YOUR ARTHRITIS

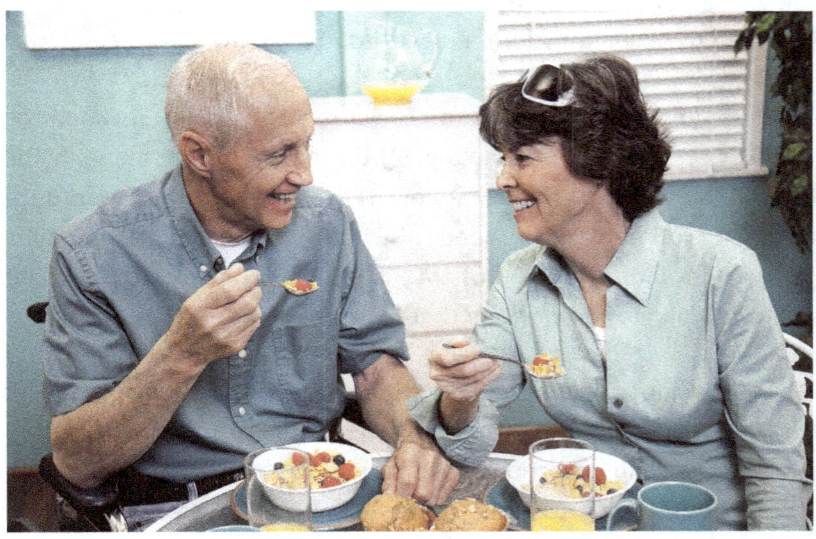

For arthritis sufferers, pain becomes a fixture in their life. Prescriptions and over-the-counter medications do provide relief, but are usually short lived. As soon as the medication wears off, the pain returns.

There is hope though. For many, that hope comes in the form of natural and dietary supplements. Just a sample of the supplements that can provide relieve include devils claw, ginger, stinging nettle, flax, and ASU.

You now know that some herbal and dietary supplements can provide arthritis relief. Your first thought may be to run to the drug store. However, before you run out and make your purchase, there a number of things you should know about these supplements.

Some herbal, dietary, and natural supplements counteract with over-the-counter and prescribed medications. For that reason, medical advice is strongly advised. Talk to a medical professional.

This should be a primary care physician or at least a pharmacist. The goal of supplements is to relieve arthritis pain and discomfort, not create other complications. If you are worried about discouragement, don't ask if a supplement will work. Instead, ask if it is safe to take with your medications.

Remember there is no cure. You can treat arthritis, but it cannot be cured. For that reason, stay away from any supplements with the claim. You will waste your money. These supplements can reduce the pain, inflammations, sleep difficulties, and decreased mobility associated with arthritis, but that is it. Plenty of products outright state this; do not opt for one that lies.

These herbal supplements are not worth putting your health at risk. As previously stated, some supplements counteract with over-the-counter and prescribed medication. If you are in severe pain, you may be willing to make the switch. You may stop taking your diabetes medication to take devils claw, and so forth. This is not recommended. Never stop taking prescribed medication. Once again, speak to a healthcare professional. Many supplements provide relief and are safe to take. Your doctor can advise you on which supplements are best.

A world of information is available online. Almost fifty herbal, natural, and dietary supplements can aid in arthritis relief. Some treat joint inflammation and swelling, while others treat sleep difficultly, decreased mobility, cartilage damage, and pain. Which is right for you? An online internet search will tell. Read reviews to see what people have to say. Look for both positive and negative reviews. It is rare for a product to receive rave reviews, but be cautious of telltale signs, such as "scam," "waste of money," or "too many side effects."

Speaking of the side effects, know what they are. Then, make an informed decision. Arthritis sufferers should examine the risk to determine if they are worth it. For example, cats claw is a supplement used to reduce inflammation. Possible side effects include headaches, vomiting, and dizziness. If your job requires you to be on your feet all day, the dizziness may be too much to handle. Look for an arthritis helping supplement that has little to no side effects.

You can and should find the best deals. In terms of supplements, the best deal isn't always the lowest price. Look for the best quality for the lowest price. This is where the above mentioned research comes in handy. Look for specific brand names with positive feedback. When buying online, compare the size with prize and include the cost of shipping.

You must follow all directions. Herbal supplements are typically safe to use, when taken as directed. Different brands use similar extracts, but those amounts vary. Consult with your primary care physician or the bottle to get an exact dosage. Despite the common belief, more will do no good. In fact, it may cause complications.

Finally, if you take herbal supplements on a daily basis, write down which ones you are taking and keep this list close to your phone or in a highly visible place like your refrigerator or bulletin board. Also, inform someone close to you. In the event you need medical care and cannot speak for yourself, responding personnel must know all medications you are taking, including supplements.

As always, you should consult with your doctor or a healthcare professional before beginning any type of treatment including using over-the-counter pain medication or supplements.

Chapter 7- Natural Remedy in Treating Arthritis

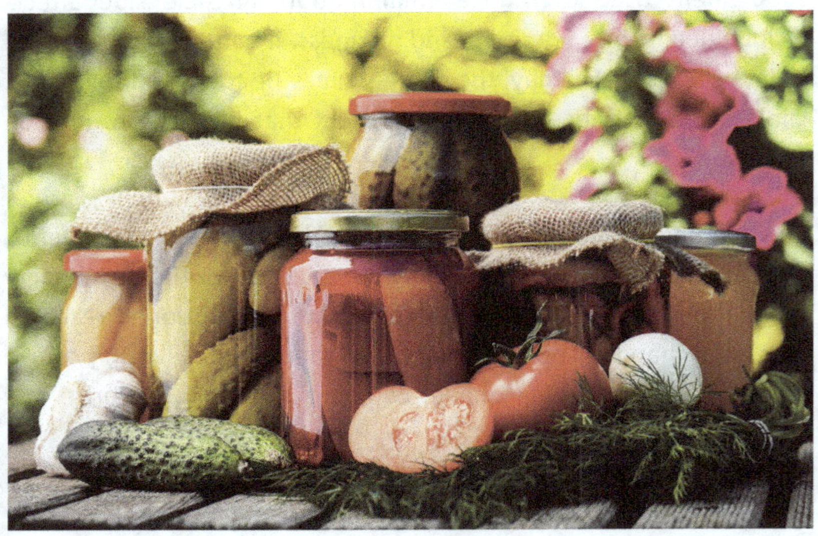

Arthritis along with numerous other conditions is now so common, they could almost be labelled as diseases of our time, and our modern world has accelerated our poor health.

Tens of millions are reported to be afflicted with one type of arthritis or another, while millions more suffer in silence. The number of known cases of arthritis has almost doubled in the last 20 years, and only seems to gather to gather momentum by the day.

It's estimated that one in three of us will experience symptoms of arthritis to some degree, at some point in our lives.

This terrible disease shows no sign of slowing, & some experts have reportedly gone as far as saying that future generations may all be affected by arthritis to some degree.

The following list of herbs, spices & roots are a combination of tried and tested tips used by thousands of RA sufferers to relieve their condition.

Herbs, spices, & roots

Herbs and spices have been used to treat various diseases and ailments for thousands of years, both herbs and spices are excellent antioxidants with many contain excellent anti inflammatory properties.

Listed below are some of the best herbs and spices known to help arthritics. It may be helpful to try to incorporate some of these herbs into your everyday life. Herbs and spices should where possible be used in their natural form & taken as a tea, or added to food. The following herbs & spices are listed in order of their superior properties when used to treat arthritis.

Some herbs and spices are known to interfere with certain prescribed medications; it is therefore always wise to consult with your doctor or a professional, before introducing any of the following herbs into your diet.

Turmeric

Has long been used to treat arthritis due to its anti-inflammatory property. Turmeric is also known to contain an antioxidant that neutralizes free radicals.

Ginger

Asian & Indian have been using ginger to treat arthritis for over 2000 years due to its anti inflammatory property.

Devils Claw

Devil's Claw is native to parts of South Africa, where it is thought to have been used to treat arthritis for centuries, two active ingredients called Harpagoside and Beta sitosterol are found in devils claw which are thought to posses excellent anti-inflammatory properties.

Devil's Claw is claimed to be beneficial for treating arthritis, rheumatism, arthritis and diseases of the liver, kidneys, gallbladder and bladder.

Cats Claw

Cat's claw has been used for over 2000 years by the indigenous peoples of South and Central America to treat rheumatic disorders. Ingredients appear to act as anti inflammatory, antioxidant and anticancer agents. Cat's claw is found in the tropical jungles of South and Central America.

Research has also indicated cats claw may help in the treatment of intestinal ailments such as Crohn's disease, gastric ulcers and tumors, parasites, colitis, gastritis, diverticulitis and leaky bowel syndrome,

Cayenne Pepper

Known to support the body's immune system. Used for treating: arthritis, backache, heart disease, ulcers, indigestion, pain, psoriasis, and shingles. Use caution when introducing cayenne pepper into your diet, although it is known to benefit many arthritics, in some cases it may actually trigger symptoms.

Cloves

Can kill intestinal parasites and act as an antimicrobial agent against fungi and bacteria. Helps relieve pain, digestive problems, and antifungal, antibacterial problems. Chewing a clove once a day may be beneficial to arthritics.

Golden seal

Known to contain a powerful detoxifier.

Parsley

Commonly used as a diuretic, & to reduce inflammation, treat rheumatism & arthritis, clear toxins in the body, inhibit tumor growth, & combat urinary tract problems.

Licorice (root)

Contains phytoestrogens. Used to treat ulcers & known to have antiviral, antitumor, anti-inflammatory properties.

Do not use licorice (root) if you have high blood pressure as large doses or prolonged use may increase blood pressure.

Do not use if you retain water easily!

Chapter 8- Foods that is Bad for Your Arthritis

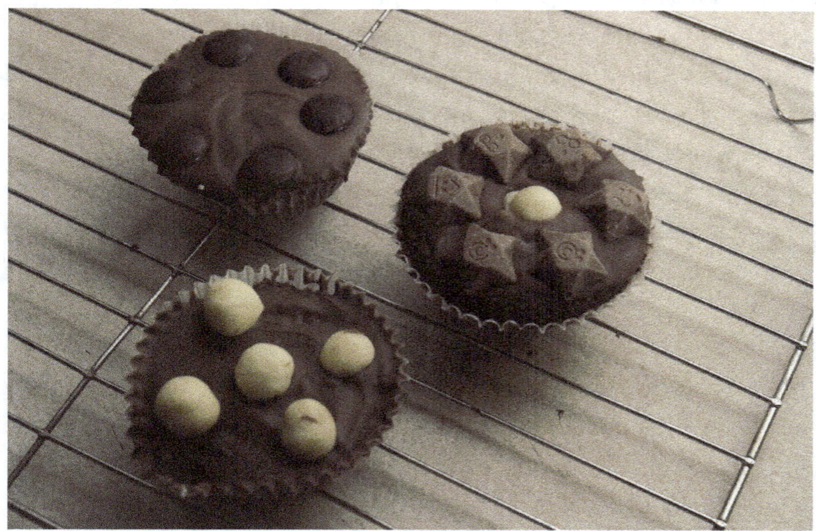

Arthritis is sometimes referred to as the 'cooked food disease.' A high combined intake of cooked, sweet, processed and fatty food can be characteristic in the development of arthritis.

Arthritis along with certain other serious diseases is more prevalent in western society. Research shows that diseases such as arthritis, cancer, heart conditions are far less common in remote or more primitive areas of the world, the reason for this is not hard to see, our industrialized, modern environment is slowly killing us all.

Rheumatoid arthritis in particular is closely linked to food allergy & intolerances. Most sufferers have been shown to greatly improve when they cut out certain foods or restrict their diet, which eliminates the foods to which they are allergic.

The food we put in our bodies can be described quite easily as either 'Good' or 'Bad.' So where do we start and what do we eat?

We shall define 'Bad' as every kind of food that is packaged, frozen, refined, processed, or otherwise changed from its natural form.

This will also include all food and produce with a long shelf life, all canned / tinned foods, all dried fruits and vegetables, all sterilized and otherwise cooked foods that are then cooled and sold in food stores, all irradiated foods, any and all junk food, etc. Candy, cakes, pies, sweets, and other such combinations are considered 'Bad.'

The following lists of foods may be of interest to those of you wishing to address their diet.

• Avoid anything containing 'Trans fatty acids' or 'Hydrogenated fat' Also known as trans fats, research has shown that trans fatty acids have many adverse effects on health, & could be responsible for increasing the risk of developing cancer, diabetes, as well as compromising the body's immune system.

• MSG 'Mono sodium glutamate is often used as a flavoring.

• All processed foods, including all junk / fast food, reformed etc.

• Alcohol

• Tinned foods

• Citrus fruits - Many arthritics have found that the acidity of citrus fruits can aggravate & trigger symptoms. Whilst in general fruits are known to have a healing potential for arthritis sufferers, experience has indicated that citrus fruits such as oranges lemons, limes and grapefruit etc., should be avoided.

- Sugar

- White, brown & all foods containing added sugar.

- Sweeteners

- Rhubarb - Arthritics should be aware that rhubarb contains a substance called oxalic acid, which can inhibit the body's ability to absorb calcium and iron from other foods.

- Salt - Except if you have low blood pressure.

- All fizzy soft drinks

- Carbonated, colas, fizzy even the diet variety.

- Coffee and tea

- And all caffeine containing beverages. - Try using green tea as an alternative, green tea contains excellent antioxidant properties.

- White rice

- Use brown as an alternative.

- Shellfish

- Fat & all fatty foods

- Fried food

- Additives and preservatives

- Mayonnaise

• Tobacco

• White flour and all foods containing white flour

• Use whole grain, and products containing whole grain as an alternative.

• All gluten containing foods,

• Gluten can damage the intestinal wall by having an irritating and inflammatory effect on the intestinal lining. Use gluten free, as an alternative.

• All foods with a long shelf life / use by date

• Dairy products

• Margarine

• Contains trans-fats or Trans fatty acids.

• Eggs

• Red meat - Especially beef and pork, Its best to remove all red meat from your diet to begin with, as many arthritics have an allergy to certain meats which may trigger an attack. You can start adding the meat back into your diet slowly and only one type of meat at a time; this will allow you to ascertain whether you have intolerance.

• Commercial breakfast cereals

• Tabasco sauce

CHAPTER 9- FOODS THAT IS GOOD FOR ARTHRITIS

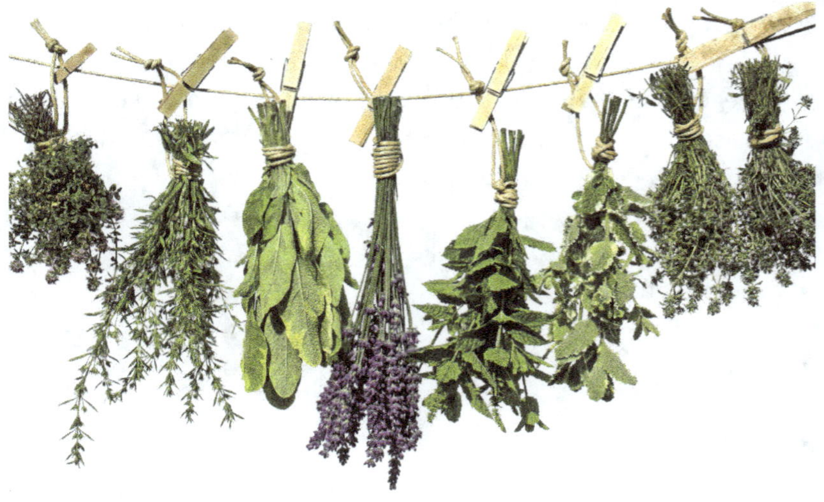

The foods which cause the most confusion amongst nutritionists and arthritis professionals are those referred to as from the nightshade family. The group of foods known as nightshade contains a substance called alkaloid which is known to have an impact on nerve and digestive function in humans and animals.

• Potatoes (especially when green and sprouting),

• Tomatoes (especially when green), Hot peppers, Sweet peppers, Paprika, Eggplant, Cayenne, Tobacco.

The amount of alkaloids contained in these foods is minimal; health problems arising from nightshade foods are rare and tend to only occur in individuals who are especially sensitive to these alkaloid substances, highly sensitive people are very likely to include arthritics.

• Good and beneficial foods

• All fruits not on the bad or caution foods list

• All root vegetables, not on the bad or caution foods list

• All vegetables that grow above ground, not on the bad or caution foods list

• Brown rice

• Sweet Potatoes

• Onions

• Garlic

• Celery

• Oily fish. Salmon, sardines, mackerel, herring. (not tinned or smoked)

• Cold water fish contain lots of Omega3 anti inflammatory oil.

• Beans Pulses

• Lamb

• Chicken & turkey (preferably organic)

• Nuts

• Except hazelnuts and peanuts

• Seeds

• Flaxseed, sunflower, pumpkins, sesame, hemp Seeds

• Green Tea - As a substitute for tea and coffee.

• Tofu and soy bean products

• As an alternative to meat.

• Berries

• All fresh berries, Especially fresh cherries, which should be eaten in abundance daily as they are known to help arthritics, most notably gout sufferers

• Fresh (real) fruit and vegetable juices

• Homemade juices are the best kind, if you have the time.

• Ginger and Turmeric (in their natural form) - Both have been used for centuries for their powerful anti-inflammatory properties.

• Olive oil (extra virgin)

• Use as an alternative to your normal cooking oil, if you do have to fry anything.

• Sea salt - Filtered water

CHAPTER 10- DON'T LET ARTHRITIS STOP YOU

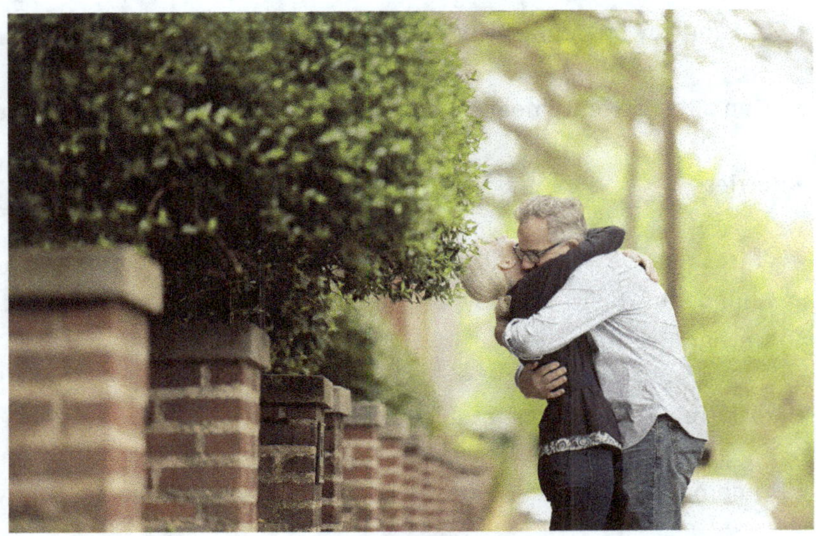

Those suffering from arthritis may find it difficult to walk to the car and back. However, most don't let arthritis stop them from enjoying their life. So, you may head out of the house and hop into your car. This is great, what if you start experiencing pain? How do you treat it on the road or prevent that pain from coming back the next time?

Keep arthritis pain relievers in the car. In one of your cars compartments, have a few pain relief supplies on hand. This may include over-the-counter pain pills, a tube of arthritis cream, or on-the-go heat patches. Whether you experience pain as soon as you get in your car, or later down the road, rely on these over-the-counter products to seek relief. If you live in an area with cold winters, do not keep these items in your car, as they may freeze. Instead, put them in your purse or fanny pack.

Speaking of over-the-counter products, most retail stores sell on-the-go heating patches. These patches stick to your body and warm with skin contact. ThermaCare is a well-known brand. They are ideal when you can't use an electric or microwaveable heating pad. If in pain before you leave the house, but must still leave, like for a holiday party or a doctor's appointment, apply an on-the-go heated patch. Relief will last for up to 12 hours. Since they stick directly to the skin, no adjustments should be needed.

Buy a remote car starter. If you live in the northern United States, it is important to warm your car first. Unfortunately, this may mean an extra trip back and forth. It doesn't have to. Instead, purchase a remote car starter. This device allows you to start and warm your car from inside your home.

They also make it easier to unlock car doors. Instead of fumbling with the keys, push the button and your car doors unlock! When buying a remote car starter, look for stores that offer free or discounted installation.

Buy no slip steeling wheel covers. Those who suffer from arthritis of the fingers, dread driving. In fact, some may fear the danger they put themselves and others in. If you find it difficult to grip your car's steering wheel, make a new purchase. That purchase should be an easy grip and slip free steering wheel cover. Ask a store employee, family member, or friend to install the cover for you.

Keep a jar opener in the car. If you have arthritis of the hands, you likely already utilize rubber jar openers at home. They make griping, twisting, and turning easier. Keep one in your car. Use it to unscrew your car's gas cap. You can also find arthritis gas cap wrenches available for sale. They slip over your gas cap, have an extended and easy grip handle. These are nice, but they can be hard to find. For the same price, you could easily buy 20 rubber jar openers, which accomplish the same goal.

Keep your car well gassed. As previously stated, there are tools available to make opening and closing the gas cap easier. Even with these tools, it can still be difficult and painful. To prevent the onset of pain, always have a full tank of gas in your car. You won't be forced to put gas in when you are already in pain or more susceptible to it. If you have a full-service gas station in your area, use it.

Just because you suffer from arthritis and are prone to pain, it does not mean you need to live your life in fear. Just take the proper precautions to reduce and prevent painful symptoms and you should have no problem staying safe on the road.

When it comes to treating the pain, stiffness, and discomfort associated with arthritis, most medical professionals recommend pain relievers and anti-inflammatory drugs. These do work, but you may be concerned with what you are putting in your body. You may want to turn to natural remedies or relief options, but are they right for you? In most cases yes, but know they do have their pros and cons.

The Pros

Your options. The phrase natural arthritis relief encompasses many different items. It all depends on your take. For example, natural supplements have all natural ingredients. But, since they are bought and sold at stores, you may not consider them a natural way to seek relief. Certain actions are also natural ways to relieve arthritis pain and discomfort.

For example, there is exercise. Those with rheumatoid arthritis have trigger factors that bring on pain. Some experience pain with strenuous joint use, others do so with certain foods. So, eating or avoid certain foods is another way to seek natural arthritis relief. Virtually, your options are endless.

Most are safe. Since these remedies are natural, if anything needs to be ingested or applied to the skin, it is all natural. This means it was found in the environment. Since there are no guarantees, caution is still advised. For example, cayenne pepper is known for the presence of capsaicin. This is also found in many overthecounter arthritis creams. Although natural, it can interact with certain medications.

Many are cheap and some are even free! For example, exercise can be free. Exercise is important because it strengths the muscles surrounding the joints. It provides extra support and protection, which should result in less pain. You can pay for a gym membership. Instead, walk around your neighborhood or stretch at home. In terms of all natural supplements and foods, look for sales, use coupons, and shop at stores known for their everyday low prices.

The Cons

There are no guarantees. Our bodies process food differently. Some arthritis patients claim eating raw cabbage or drinking cabbage juice reduces arthritis pain and inflammation. On the other hand, it does nothing for others. In fact, some cannot stomach the taste and others are allergic! Your best option is to familiarize yourself with popular natural remedies and then experiment to find the best form of relief for your own body.

Arthritis Cure: Natural Ways to Beat Arthritis

Some natural remedies require prolonged use. Research apple cider vinegar and arthritis online. You will find a ton of remedies and information on how it does work. With that said, you will also see that prolonged use is required. Some patients stop drinking apple cider vinegar mixtures or stop soaking their body due to the reduction in pain and swelling. Many are disappointed to later see the pain and inflammation return.

Some natural remedies can get costly, especially overtime. You just heard that continued use is best for maximum and long-term relief of pain and swelling. Unfortunately, this means you need to buy more.

Remember, exercise is free. As for heat, opt for a warm bath. If you need to use a heating pad, save the onetime patches for on-the-go use. At home, use a reusable heating pad. In short, natural remedies do have their pros and cons, but there is no way to know what will work unless last you try.

About the Author

Judith Peters suffered arthritis during her early twenties. She can't believe then that such a young age she is a victim of this incurable disease. But that didn't stop Judith to educate herself about her condition.

Her condition led her to devote years of systematically researching and educating herself on how to go about overcoming her illness. She compiled all the information that she gathered and put it in a book so she may be able to help others who are suffering with this kind of illness.

She now lives an active lifestyle in Florida with her family.